Friends
All Around

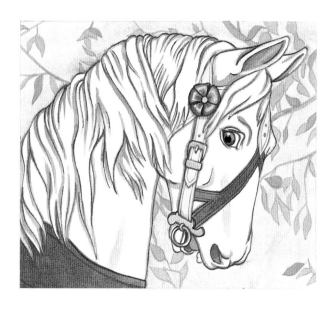

By JoAnne Nelson
Illustrated by Tracy duCharme

Published by
The Wright Group
19201 120th Avenue NE
Bothell, WA 98011-9512

©1995 by Comprehensive Health Education Foundation (C.H.E.F.®)
22323 Pacific Highway South
Seattle, WA 98198

Printed in Canada.

99 98 97 96 95   5 4 3 2 1

Library of Congress Cataloging-in-Publication Data
Nelson, JoAnne
        Friends All Around/by JoAnne Nelson; Illustrated by Tracy duCharme.
        p.   cm.
        Summary: Children on a class outing to an amusement park enjoy interacting with their
        disabled friends, one of whom is deaf, one blind, one with Down's syndrome, and one
        in a wheelchair.
        [Physically handicapped — Fiction. 2. Mentally handicapped — Fiction.
        3. Merry-go-round — Fiction. 4. Amusement parks — Fiction.] I. duCharme, Tracy, ill., II. Title.
        P27.n4344Fr   1992   [E] — dc20

ISBN: 0-7802-3243-7   CIP 92-4657
ISBN: 0-7802-3098-1 (6-pack)

Sara, Sara, come and play.
We're going to the park today!

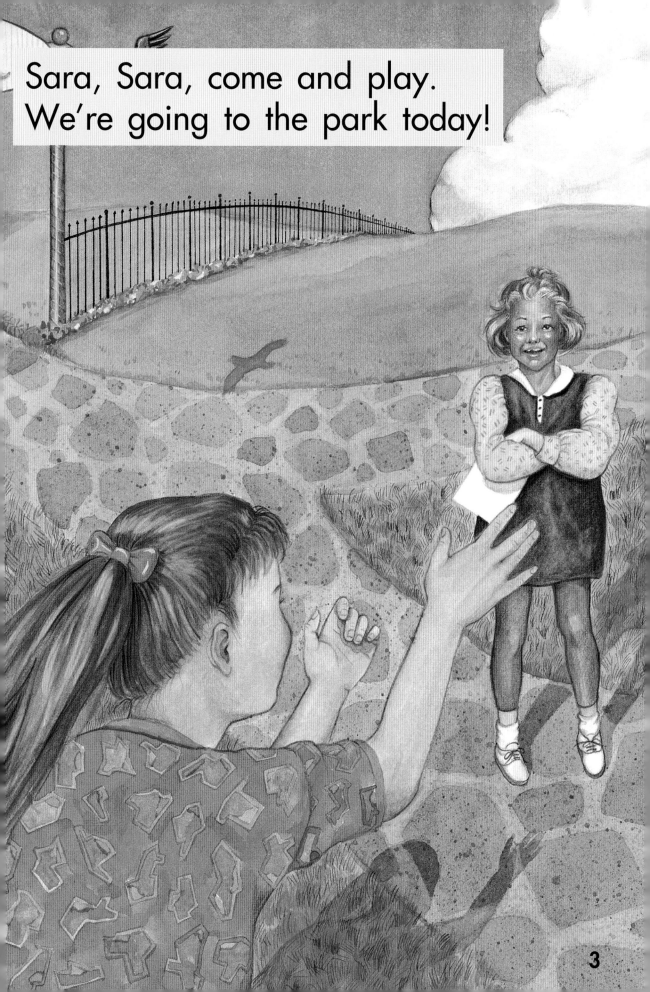

Sara can't hear my voice,
so we talk with signing.
Sara is my best friend.

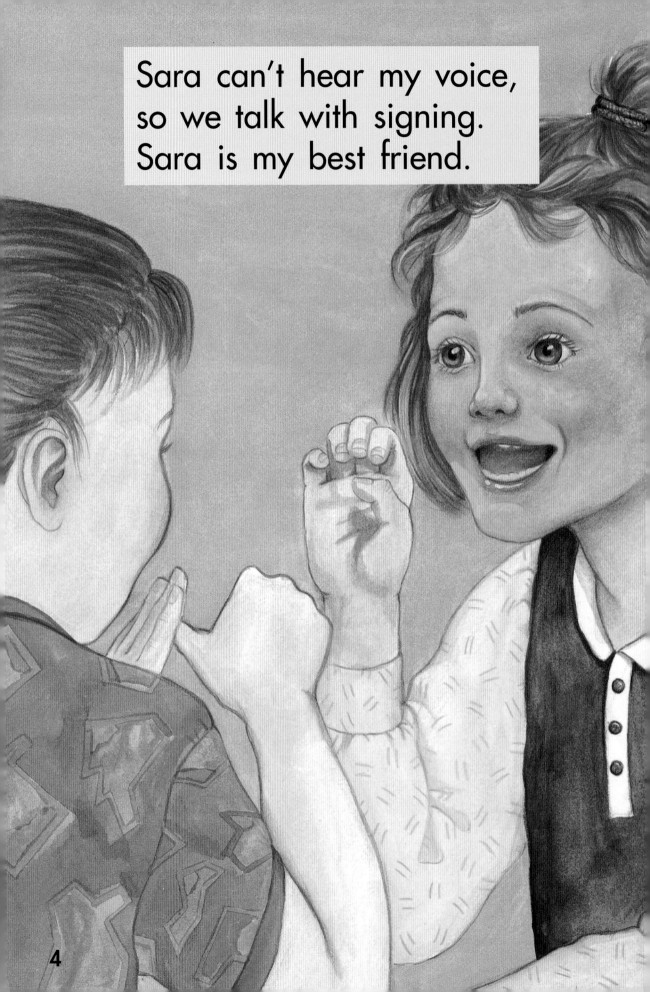

Sara can't hear the music,
but she can feel the movements
and vibrations.
Sara smiles because she loves
to ride on the merry-go-round.

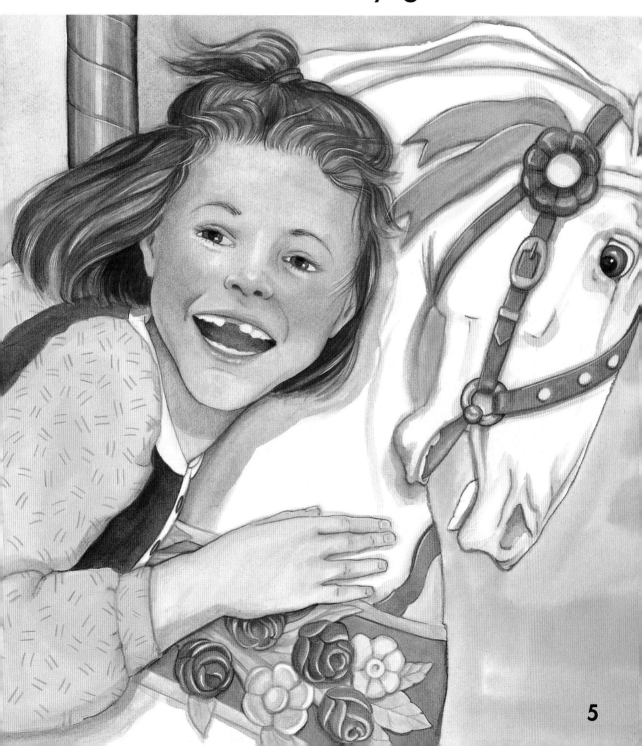

When I first met Sara,
she almost got hit by a bicycle
because she couldn't hear
the rider shouting.

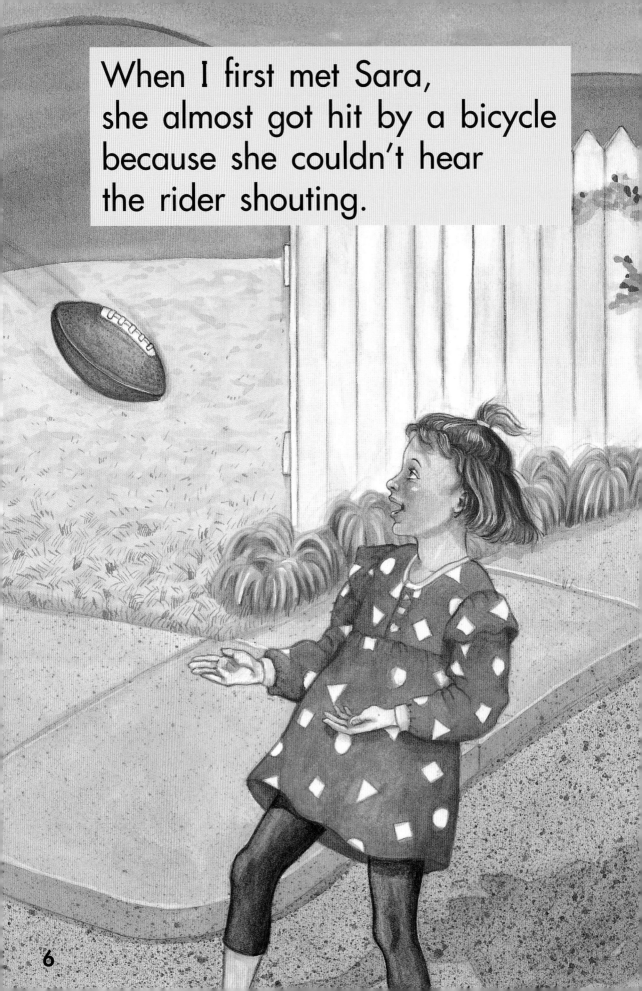

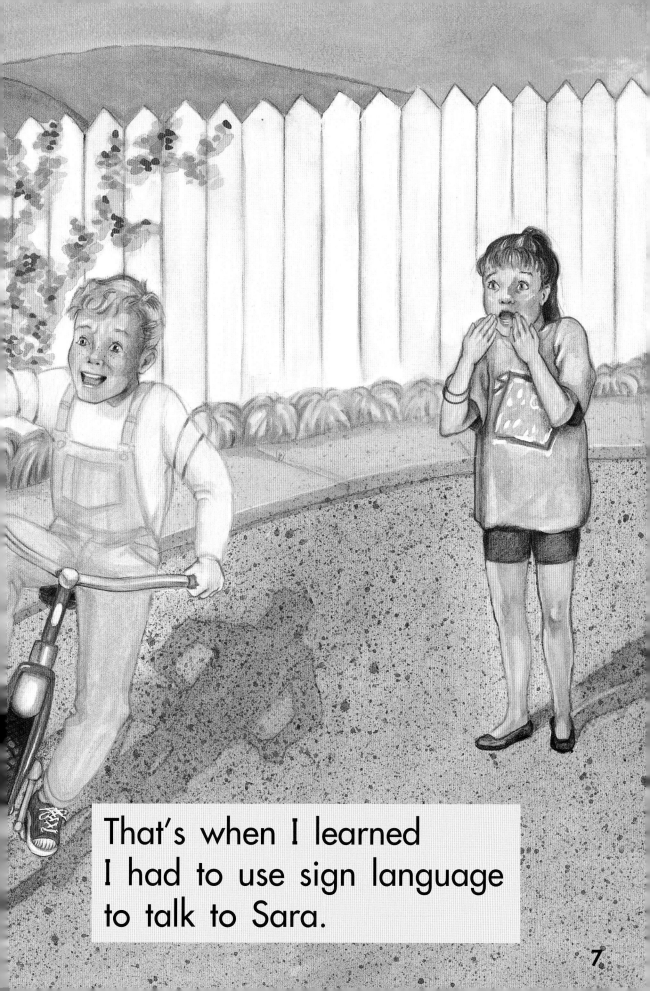

That's when I learned
I had to use sign language
to talk to Sara.

Andrew, Andrew, come with me.
The merry-go-round is fun—
you'll see!

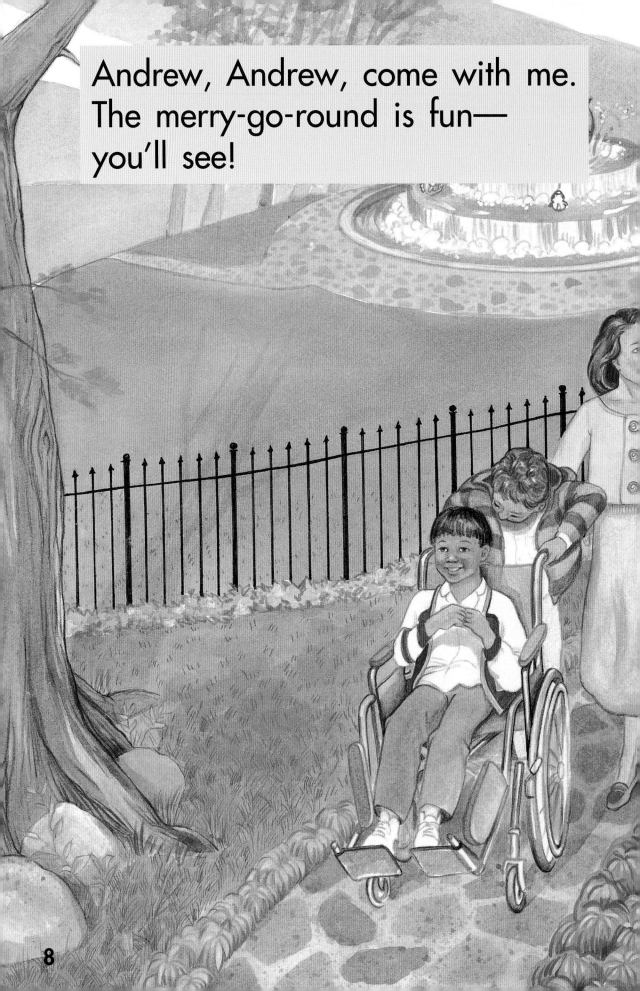

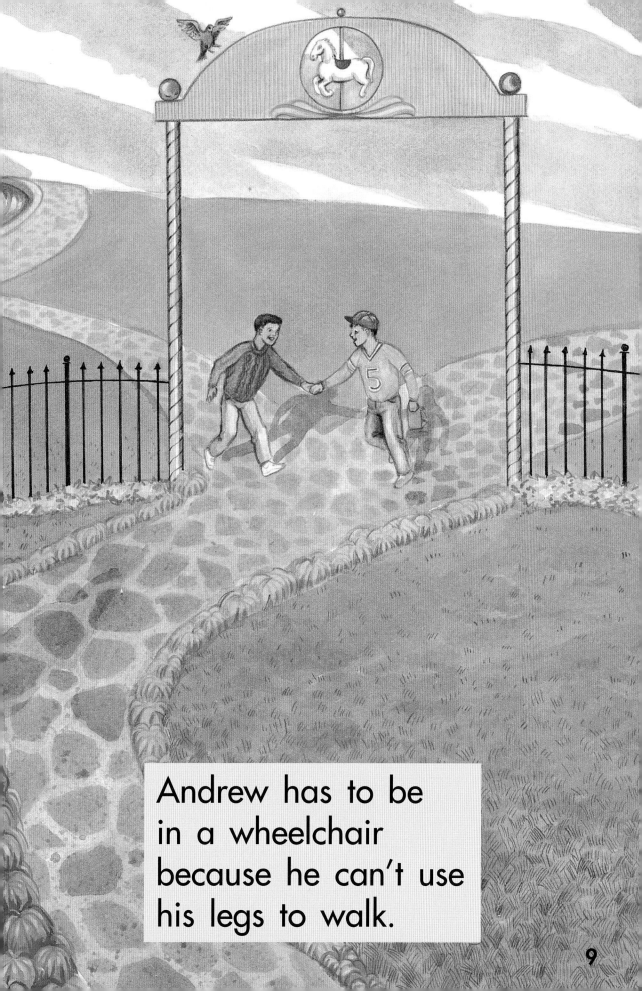

Andrew has to be
in a wheelchair
because he can't use
his legs to walk.

Andrew's wheelchair can't go on the merry-go-round, but we can help him get on.

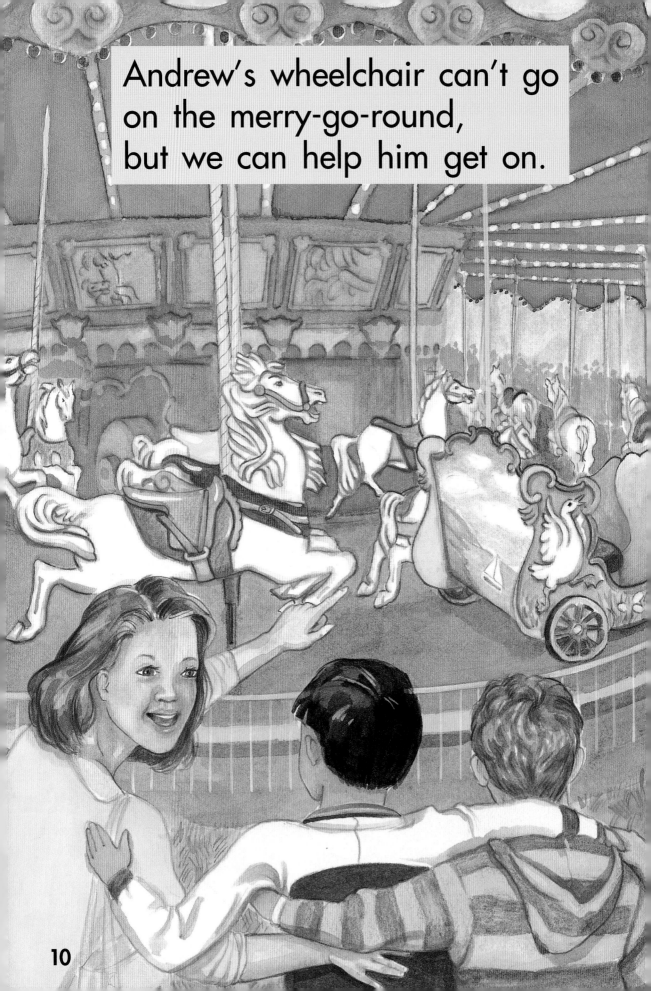

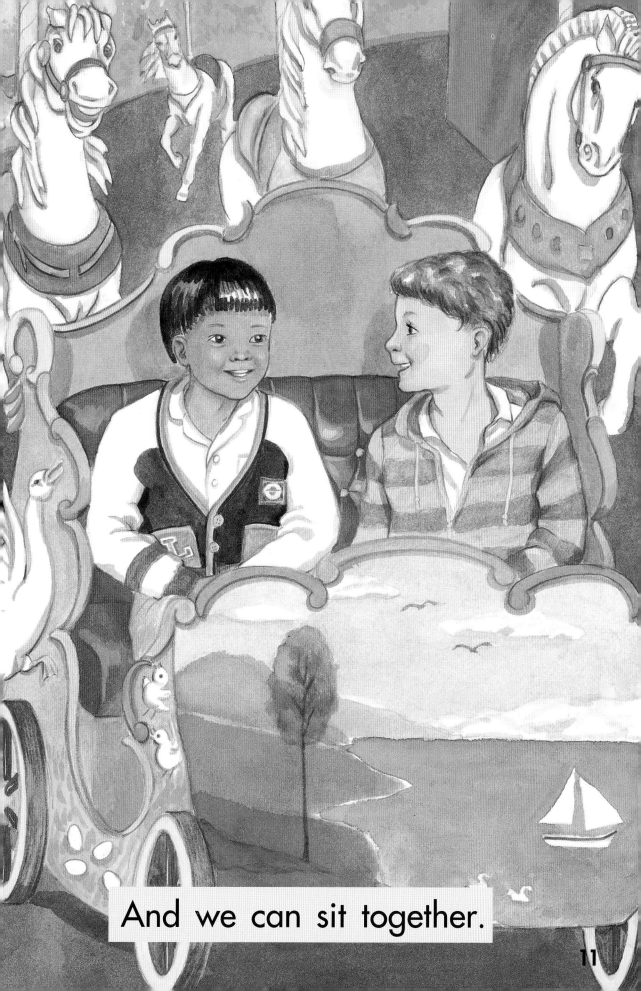

And we can sit together.

When I first met Andrew,
he was in a swim meet.
That's when I learned
that Andrew's arms are strong.

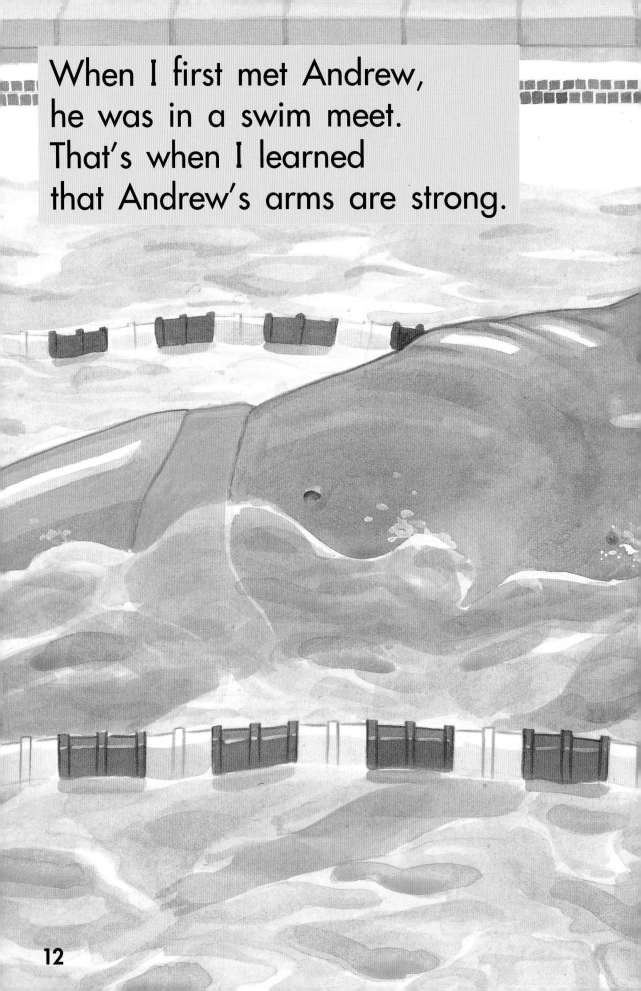

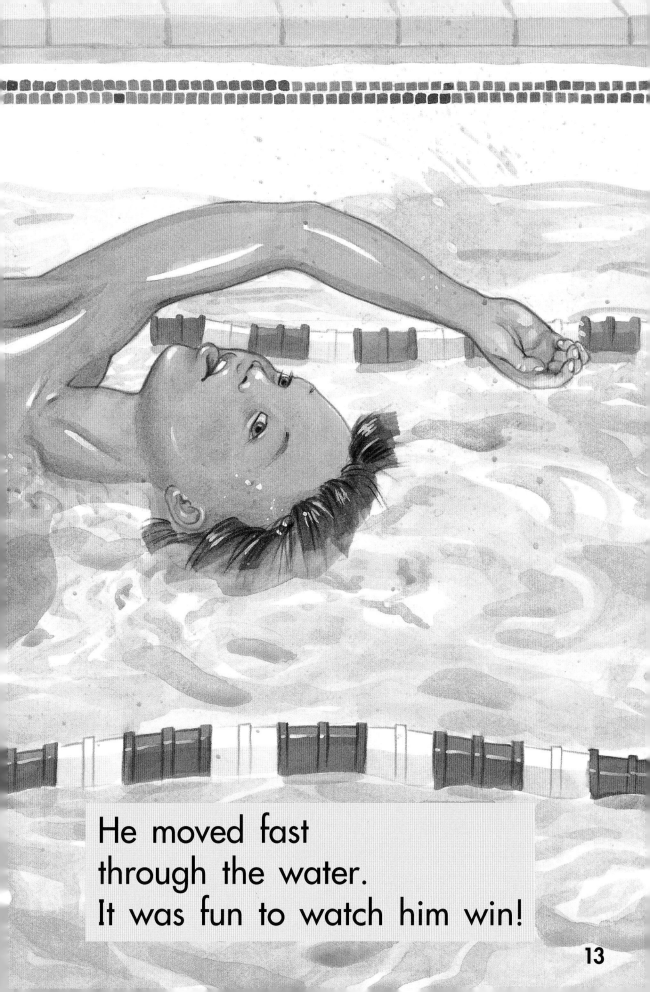

He moved fast
through the water.
It was fun to watch him win!

Laura, Laura, hear the sound,
and feel the horse go up and down!

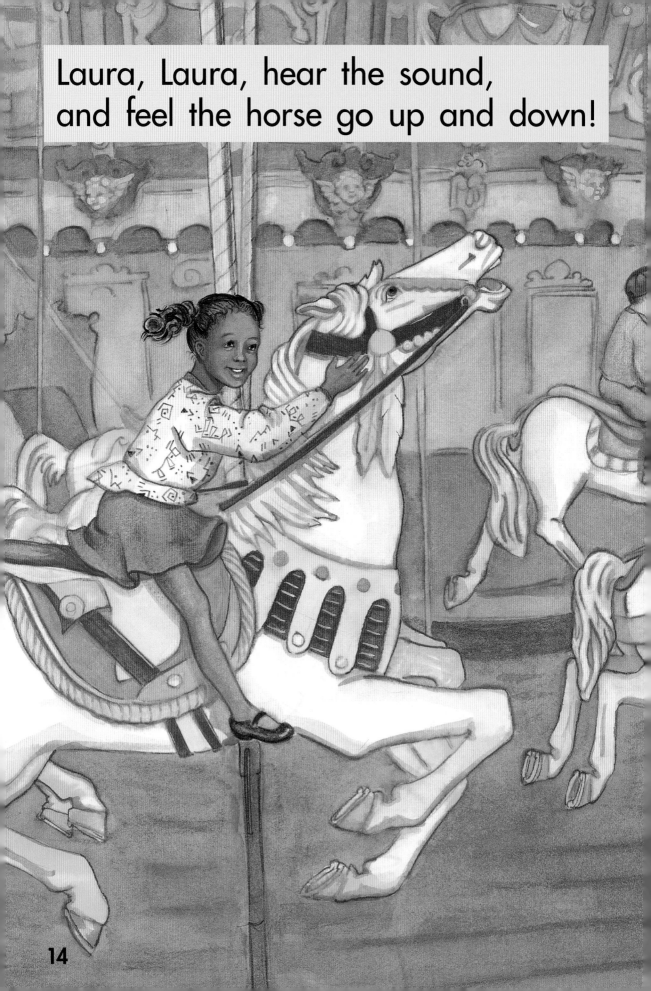

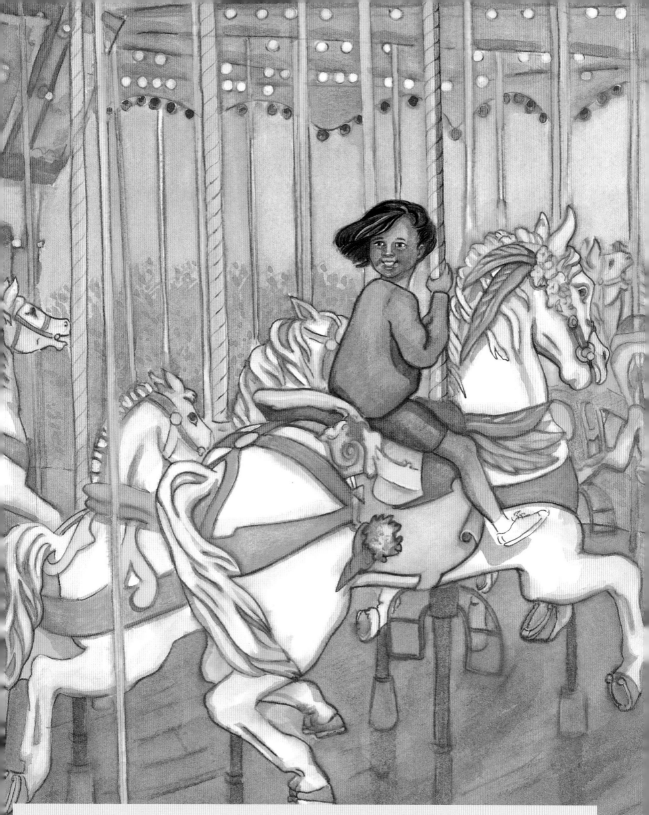

Trace the horse's head and mane
while we hold on tight.
Laura, can you feel the wind?

Even though Laura is blind, she can see light and dark and some shapes.

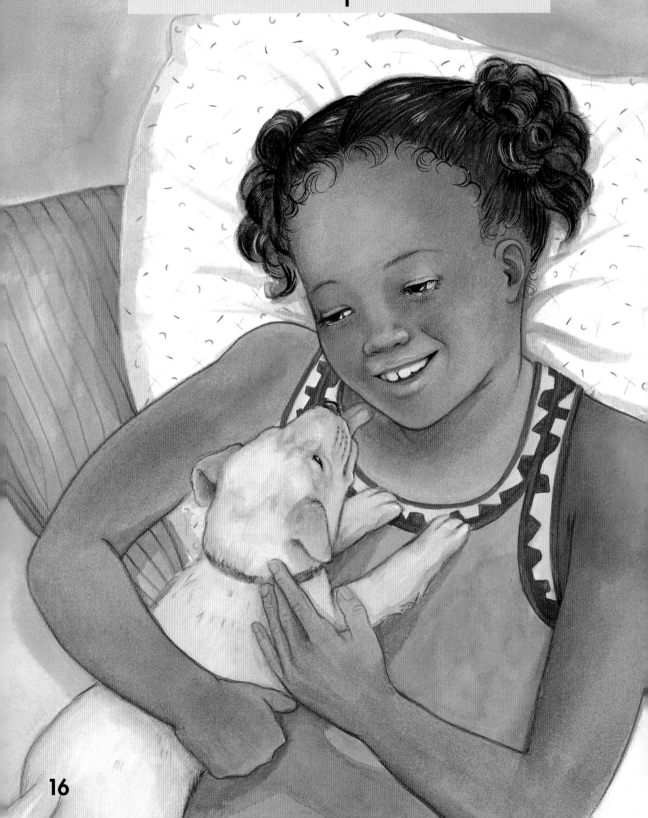

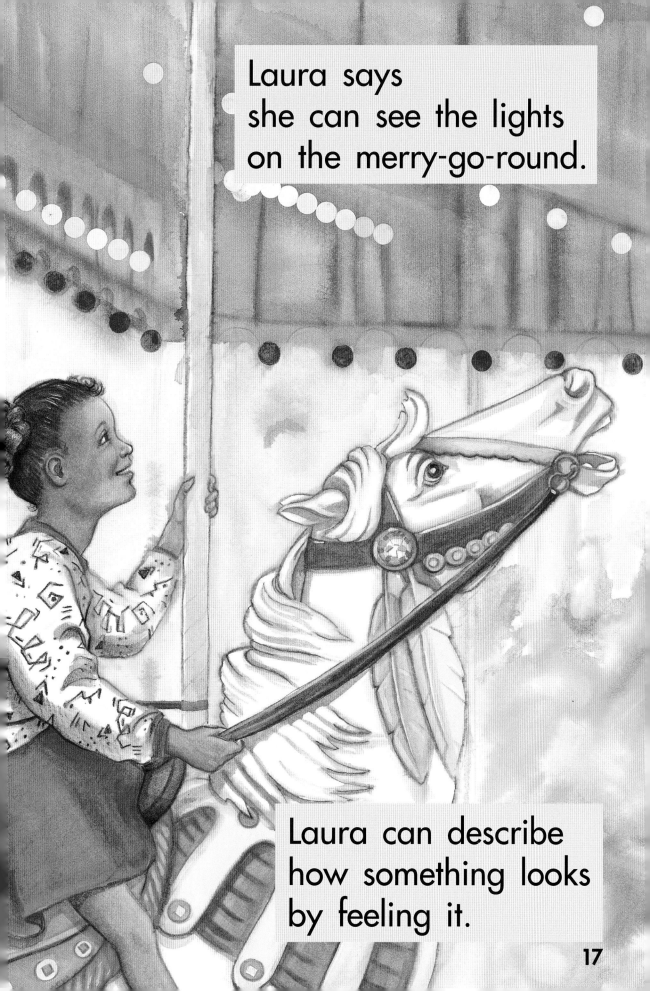

Laura says
she can see the lights
on the merry-go-round.

Laura can describe
how something looks
by feeling it.

Laura can read her name, too.
I remember the day she taught me
how to read by touching.
It was like reading a secret code.

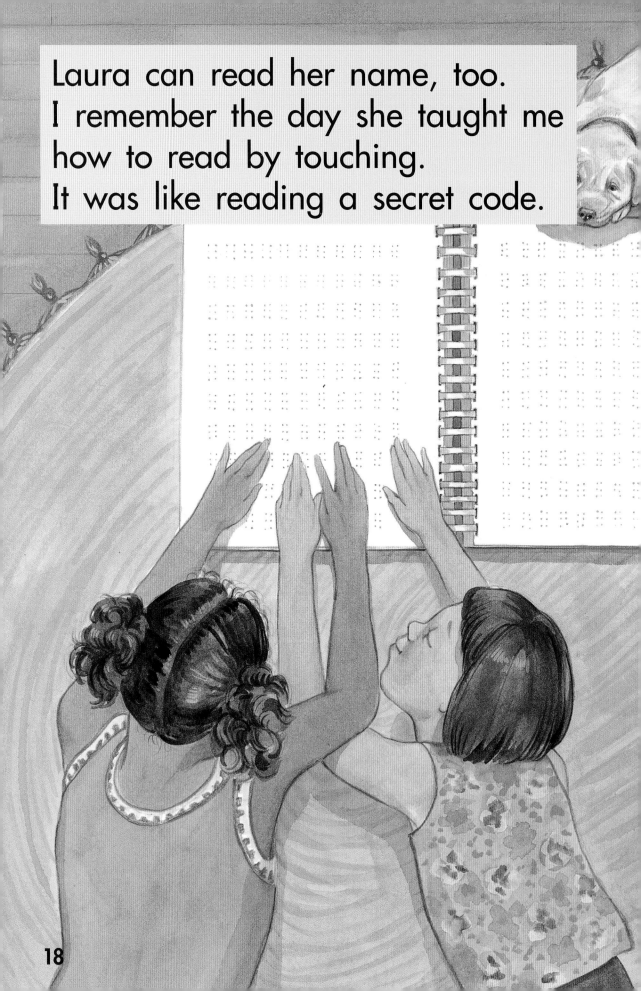

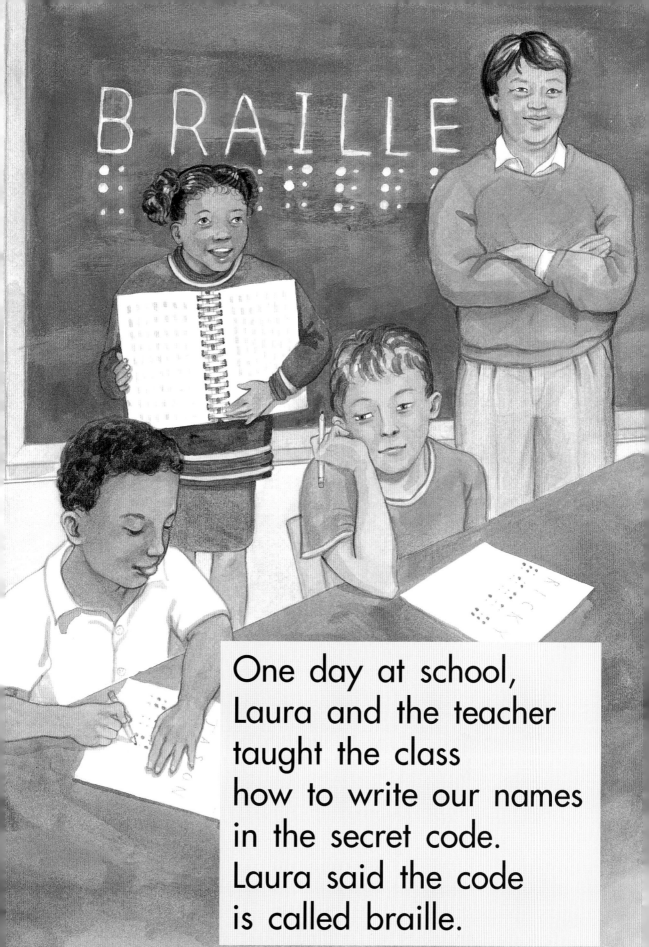

One day at school,
Laura and the teacher
taught the class
how to write our names
in the secret code.
Laura said the code
is called braille.

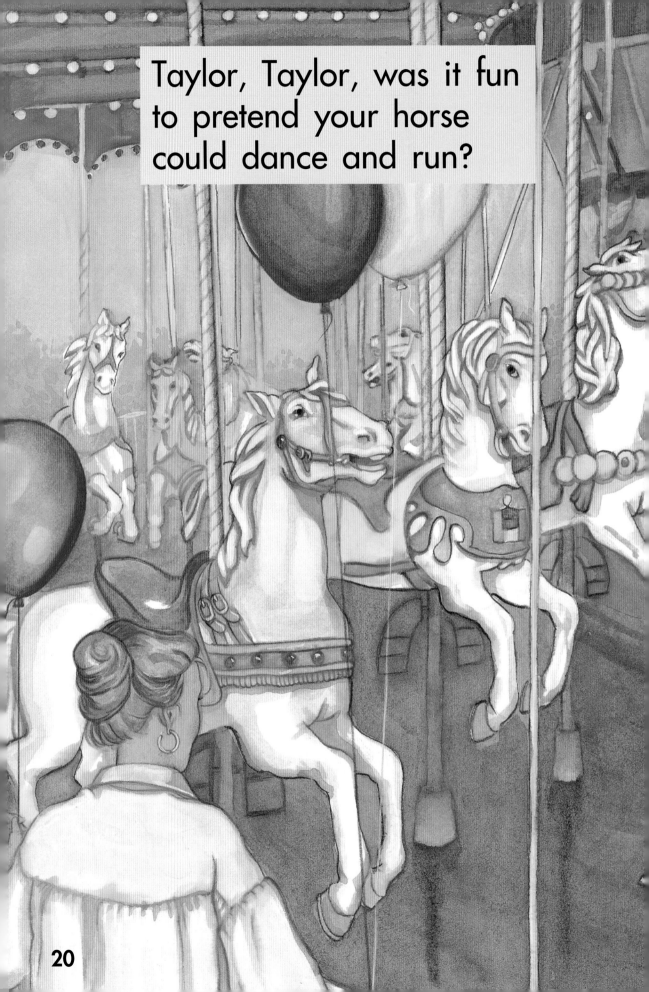

Taylor, Taylor, was it fun to pretend your horse could dance and run?

20

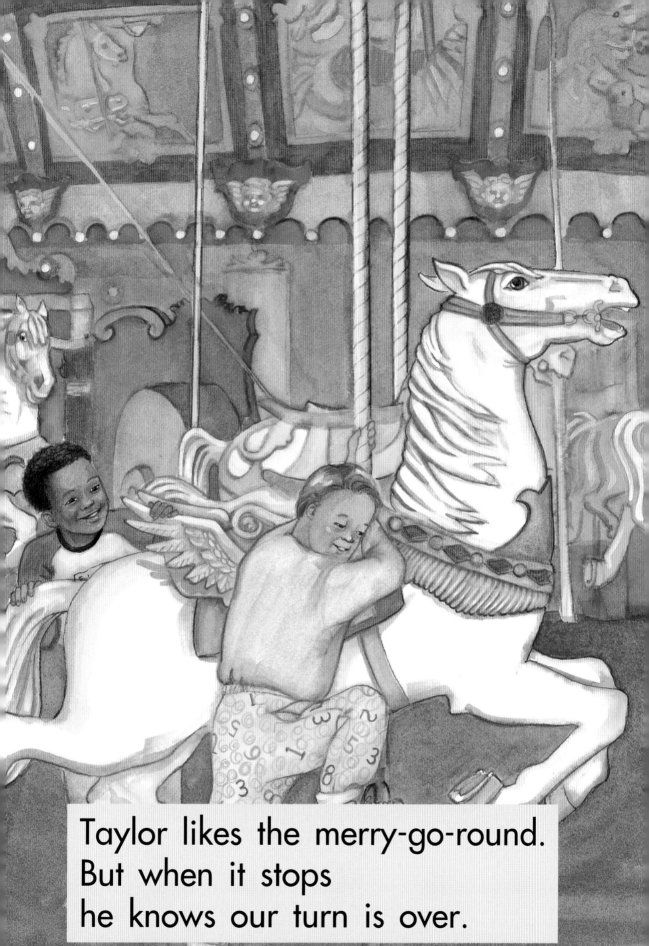

Taylor likes the merry-go-round.
But when it stops
he knows our turn is over.

Taylor likes to help
pass out the lunches.
Then we find a shady spot
to sit and eat together.

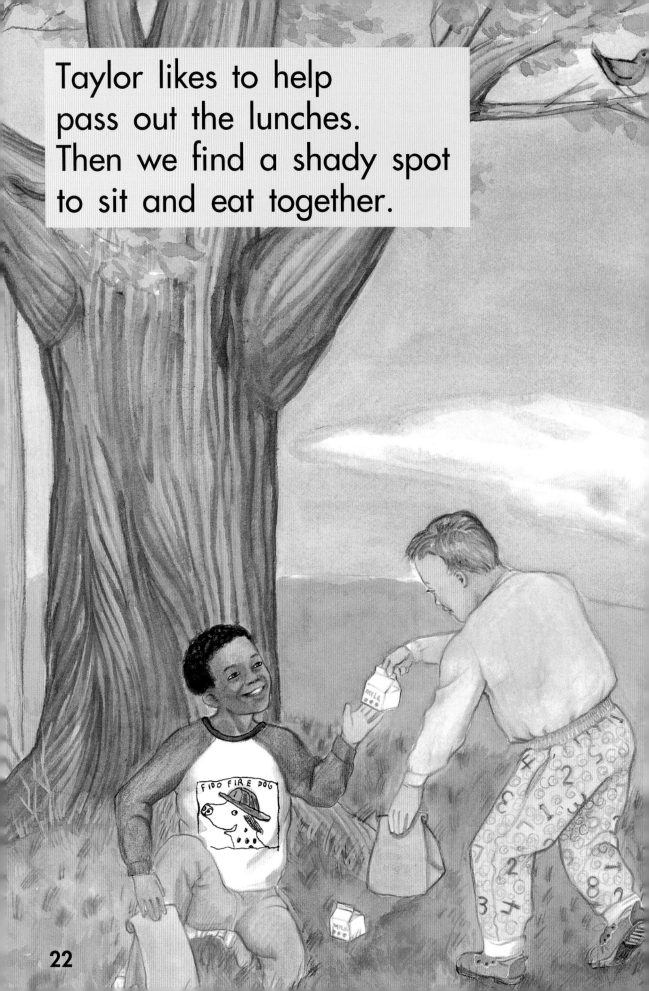

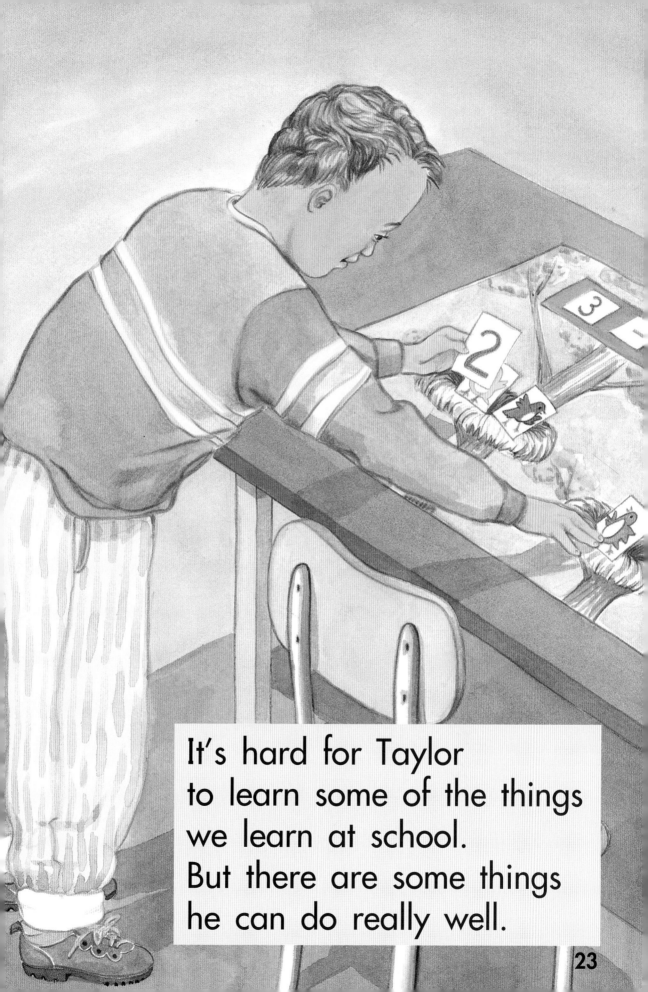

It's hard for Taylor
to learn some of the things
we learn at school.
But there are some things
he can do really well.

When we're at the park,
at school, or at play,
we're friends all around.
We like it that way!

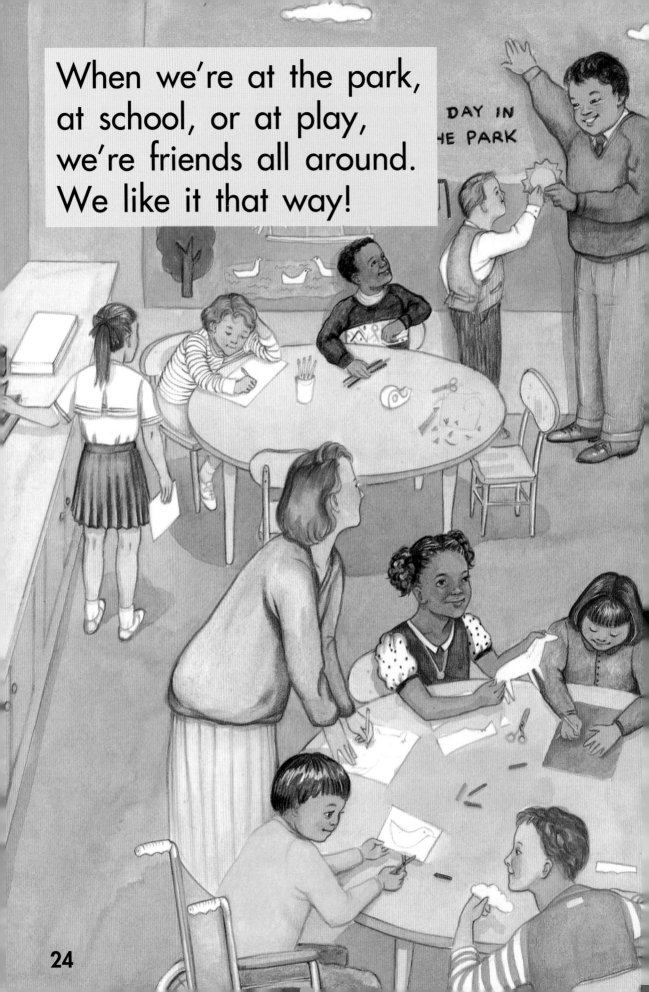